World's Most Powerful Dog Cancer Treatment

Cure your dog's cancer simply, cheaply in as little as 90 days in 3 easy steps

By: Diana Gordon

for the Canine Research Foundation

Copyright

DISCLAIMER **4**

INTRODUCTION **6**

A SECOND CHANCE 10
HOW ONE PET OWNER REVERSED HER DOG'S CANCER BY DISOBEYING HER
VET 12

THE FIRST RULE **16**

#1 ELIMINATE DAMAGING FATS AND FOOD 16

THE SECOND RULE **24**

SUPER CHARGE YOUR DOG'S HEALTH 24
WORLD'S MOST POWERFUL ANTI-OXIDANT 27
ASTAXANTHIN STUDY WITH BEAGLES 28
How much astaxanthin should you give your dog? 28
GREEN TEA 30
ARGININE L 32
CATS CLAW 33
ENZYMES 34
COENZYME Q10 35
OMEGA 3 FATTY ACIDS 36
MILK THISTLE 38
A SUPERFOOD FOR DOGS 40
MARY NEVER GAVE UP ON TED 41

THE THIRD RULE **44**

OXYGENATE CELLS WITH THE "POWER MIX" 44
MAKING THE MIX 49
How to tell if this Protocol is working 52
IMPORTANT INFORMATION ABOUT FLAX OIL 53
How to Feed our Dog after they are Cured 55
MORE TIPS TO BOOST YOUR DOG'S IMMUNE SYSTEM 59
THE TRUTH ABOUT CHEMOTHERAPY 60

REFERENCES **63**

DISCLAIMER

The following is meant for informational purposes only. Please consult a holistic veterinarian before making any changes to your dog's treatment plan.

INTRODUCTION

What you're about to hear is the untold story of how cancer, under the right circumstances, can be defeated.

My name is Diana Gordon.

I never expected to publish a book on beating Cancer.

I stumbled on the 90 Day Canine Cancer Miracle by accident...

While researching human cures for a famous natural medicine doctor in Florida.

At the time, I lived with a friend and her four dogs, three who were struck by tumors. Despite veterinary visits and surgeries, all three passed away.

Not long later, my best friend lost her dog Juniper to cancer.

It was then that I began to wonder, why are so many dogs getting cancer? What is causing it? Has anyone discovered a cure?

During my quest for an answer, a colleague told me about the 90 Day Canine Cancer Miracle.

I was floored.

Could this really cure more than 90% of cancer cures?

The treatment you're about to see was discovered by a five time Nobel Prize nominee, Dr. Johanna Budwig. Not a charlatan or a quack, but an expert in several fields such as pharmacology, physics, and chemistry. Dr. Budwig made her cancer curing discovery in 1951. Today, her discoveries are still held in high regard in Germany and neighboring countries.

Still, I was skeptical.

Why didn't more Americans know about this cure?

If it could eradicate cancer, why wasn't it splashed on the front page of every newspaper?

So I decided to get answers.

I contacted Lloyd Alexander, who ran the Budwig Clinic in Spain. He worked directly with Dr. Johanna Budwig before she passed away in 2003 to discover how to use the 90 Day Canine Cancer Miracle you're about to see.

He told me story after story of incurable cancer CURED… and all the proof was in black and white on his website.

Including pictures, names, and information submitting by the patients cured.

After several calls and emails, I flew to the clinic to see exactly how cancer patients were healed.

What I saw blew my mind.

And is the foundation of the book you're about to read.

Although it is easy to laugh at the simplicity of this book or write it off as junk because the powerful, 90-day treatment is packed into a few, short pages, the proof that this miracle works is overwhelming.

If your dog is sick or you know of a dog owner suffering from canine cancer, you need to try the 90 Day Canine Cancer Cure Immediately.

It could be the most important thing you do this year.

Because whatever you've been told, cancer is not a death sentence.

There are simple natural cures people don't want you to find out about.

Because they threaten the livelihood of millions of people in the cancer industry.

As Johanna Budwig famously proclaimed…

"I have the answer to cancer, but American doctors won't listen. They come here and observe my methods and are impressed. Then they want to make a special deal so they can take it home and make a lot of money. I won't do it, so I'm blackballed in every country."

And from Johanna's cure, thousands of dogs, just like yours, have found relief from cancer.

My hope for you is that you will find the answers to cancer you are looking for, and give your dog a second chance at life.

But before I go on I want to make one thing clear…

I'm not a doctor or scientist…

I can't diagnosis your dog or give you any specific recommendations.

But what I can do is give you the full details on some astonishing treatments for canine cancer that are rarely covered in the mainstream news or recommended by Veterinarians.

Treatments that prove cancer has been successfully eradicated time and time again.

And while these remedies are not magic and there are no guarantees…they give your dog the very best chance of beating canine cancer.

Everything you're about to hear is grounded in rock solid science.

Now I know first-hand how terrifying it is to receive a diagnosis from your Vet but I'm here to tell you if you're willing to follow the steps in this simple guide, you can experience a miracle.

What's more, the material you're about to receive is not paid for by a fancy publishing house or some high minded academic journal, there is no agenda to push, and no great profit to be made.

In fact, it took three years and tens of thousands of dollars to deliver to you.

So, if you've gotten that terrible diagnosis about your best friend…take heart. The solutions you're about to hear have healed and fixed countless cancer cases.

Much like Gabby.

A Second Chance

Gabby lay on the kitchen floor exhausted. Her eyes were dull and lifeless.

She had barely moved in two days.

As you can see from the mound on Gabby's nose in this picture, Gabby had incurable cancer. Her veterinarian had written her off as dead.

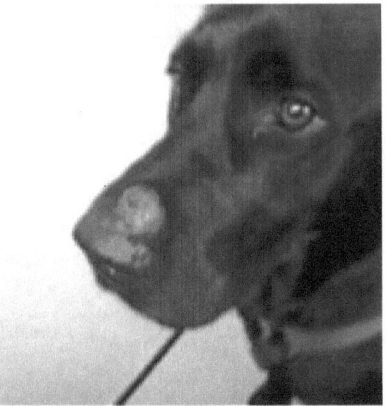

Yet, just 90 days later, Gabby was jumping around the yard, barking and full of life. Her tumor was gone for good.

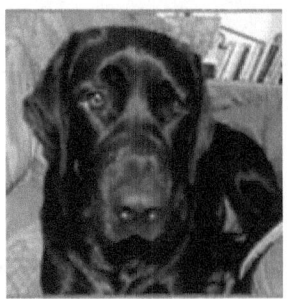

That was a decade ago.

Today, Gabby is cancer free. A miracle? Perhaps. But Science is proving otherwise. Today, thousands of dogs are beating cancer as you'll see in a moment.

What caused Gabby's remarkable change and the change in thousands of dogs just like her?

How was it that Gabby's cancer disappeared, without chemotherapy and without drugs, when the vast majority of all cancer cases end fatally?

The answer will surprise you.

How One Pet Owner Reversed Her Dog's Cancer by Disobeying Her Vet

Sarah was told Gabby had no chance to live. That's why Sarah set out on a quest to cure Gabby herself. And that's when Sarah stumbled on an amazing natural cure.

A cure that was first discovered by German scientists before WWII, and kept largely in the shadows for years after.

According to major university studies, this cure does something no other human or animal treatment does for dogs. It starves cancer cells to death.

How?

By simply "FEEDING" your dog's cells the right combination of oils and proteins you can starve cancer cells right out of your dog's body.

If this sounds hard to believe, we're on the same page. I was skeptical at first too until I saw the research.

It all starts back in 1931, when German physiologist and medical doctor Otto Heinrich Warburg discovered the true cause of cancer.

Look at how he addressed a prestigious gathering of Nobel Laureates:

> *"Cancer, above all other diseases, has countless secondary causes. But, even for cancer, there is only one prime cause. Summarized in a few words, the prime cause of cancer is the replacement of the respiration of oxygen in normal body cells by a fermentation of sugar."*

What does that mean?

Well, what Dr. Otto Warburg (who would go on to receive the Nobel Prize in 1931) was saying was that when cells can no longer absorb oxygen, cancer can develop.

In other words ...

"The Lack of Oxygen in cells is the #1 Cause of Cancer."

Without oxygen, cancer takes over. Cell functions shut down. Normal bodily functions like eating, urinating and even breathing become increasingly difficult.

According to Warburg, *"It is indisputable that all cancer could be prevented if the respiration of body cells were kept intact."*

Said another way, if you can oxygenate your dog's cells, you can kill cancer and block future cancer cells from forming.

Now you're probably wondering, if it's so simple, why haven't I heard about it?

As sickening as it is to think about, the answer is money.

No, your Vet is not the one to blame. They are doing the best they can with their training, and the information they are taught in Veterinary school.

The sad fact is, drugs and cancer treatment are big business in America. Because there is no money to be made in studying natural treatments, much of the breakthrough research we see on natural treatments is done outside the U.S.

And the 90 Day Canine Cancer Miracle is no different.

So, what is the cure and how do can you start using it today?

I'll show you.

The cure has to do with three rules.

When you follow them, cancer cannot exist.

Now these three rules are simple, but their results are remarkably powerful.

In the next section, I'm going to show you how to use these three rules to starve cancer, stop pain, heal your dog's joints, protect his heart, and keep him happy and sharp for years to come.

All for just a few dollars a month.

THE FIRST RULE

"Any cancer prevention or treatment program begins with diet. Nothing will go farther in promoting health than a balanced, home-prepared diet of fresh, preferably organic, whole foods."

#1 Eliminate damaging fats and food

You've probably heard some veterinarian, pet food manufacturer or someone in conversation say that grains (rice, barley, oats, etc.) are very good ingredients in cat and dog foods, are easy to digest and will give your cats and dogs "energy and vitality."

I certainly have.

But, nothing could be further from the truth.

As Los Angeles veterinarian and owner of "The Pet Print," Dr. Patrick Mahaney said,

"Our companion animals suffer life threatening toxicity thanks to certain pet food manufacturer's efforts to create a less expensive product using poorer quality ingredients."

These ingredients, of course, are grain, rice, and corn. After all, natural ingredients cost more.

The trouble is dog's digestive systems aren't' designed to digest grains and starches.

So, when they are fed a steady diet of cheap fillers and not real food, your pet's cells are starved of oxygen and cancer is given a chance to grow.

But dog food companies don't want you to know this.

Even the American Veterinary Medical Association (AVMA) recently told veterinarians to discourage pet owners from feeding raw pet food diets...

Despite pet owners reporting their dogs are the healthiest they've ever been thanks to the raw food diet.

Like veterinarian Dr. Laurie Coger, DVM who says she has been feeding her dogs an all raw diet for 20 years because it's kept her dogs noticeably healthier than her client's kibble eating dogs.

"Are we veterinarians promoting health or the dog food industry?" she says).

And Dr. Elizabeth Hodgkins calls many pet diseases "human creations" thanks to their high carbohydrate, highly processed diet.

"Grains are not needed, digestible or good for our carnivorous pets." - Dr. Jeannie Thomason, CVND

Unfortunately, most of our commercial dog foods are based on rice, wheat or corn.

So, the first rule for feeding a dog with cancer is to STAY AWAY FROM GRAINS!

Dogs did not evolve as grain eaters.

They have evolved as primarily meat eaters.

They simply do not produce the enzymes necessary to digest grains.

Read your dog food label: make sure the first ingredient on the list is some type of meat.

You will almost always find some grains listed, but they should be down the list always, not right at the top.

For example, if you must buy a commercial dog food, some grains are better than others.

Sorghum is a better filler than corn, which is better than rice or wheat.

But these foods are still missing critical nutrients your dog needs to feed his cells, like protein.

For a canine cancer case, any commercial dry food should be supplemented with additional animal protein sources.

Try adding canned sardines (best), cottage cheese, eggs and just about any kind of meat such as hamburger or ground turkey if you feed your dog dry foods.

And that brings me to another important point in healing your dog's cells. Not only does a sick canine need protein, but he also needs fats.

High-fat content is good. It oxygenates your dog's cells. So, what kind of diet is naturally high fat and high protein?

One option is the raw diet. It's become very controversial in the media
because of the possibility of bacterial contamination.

But many dogs are fed raw diets to improve their health. High-performance dogs like Greyhounds and Alaskan Huskies are fed raw diets to improve their performance.

Take the Iditarod dogs, for example.

Called "The Last Great Race on Earth," dogs race in temperatures far below zero, in winds that cause complete loss of visibility, and through treacherous climbs that require all senses firing at peak performance.

Eating the right diet could be the difference between life and death.

According to Licensed Veterinary Technician and Iditarod volunteer Jenna Herne, Iditarod dogs must eat a special blend of raw meat along with veggies and vitamins to keep them at peak performance because they run more than 1000 miles in less than 15 days (the record is eight days).

And dogs with cancer are facing a similar battle. They need to have the best diet possible because their cells are involved in a competition as grueling as the Iditarod... beating cancer.

The results aren't lost on the veterinarian community.

While there is no consensus yet, Australian veterinarian Ian Billinghurst makes a compelling case for feeding dogs his Biologically Appropriate Raw Food diet or BARF for short.

Billinghurst suggests that adult dogs will do best on an evolutionary diet based on what canines ate before they became domesticated: Raw, meaty bones and vegetable scraps. Grain-based commercial pet foods, he argues are harmful to your dog's health.

While there is some controversy because a raw food diet's bacteria level, potential benefits of the raw dog food diet include:

Shinier coats

Healthier skin

Cleaner teeth

Higher energy levels

Smaller stools

Whether you go raw or not, here's a good rule of thumb...

According to Dr. Ogilvie who worked alongside the Morris Animal Foundation, keep your dog on a diet consisting of limited quantities of simple sugars, moderate amounts of complex sugars, high-quality digestible proteins (in moderate amounts), and specific amounts of certain types of fat.

His research led to the manufacturing of Hill's Science Diet n/d which is cancer specific.

So to sum up, before you can use the 90 Day Canine Cancer Miracle, check your dog's diet for cancer feeding agents: grains and sugars...

And cut them out.

How do I know what ingredients in my dog's food are simple sugars?

Simple sugars consist of any processed sugar and fruit sugar. These would include rice syrup, molasses, honey, corn syrup, maple sugar or syrup, glucose, sucrose, and dextrose. Almost anything ending in "ose" is considered a simple sugar. More examples of simple sugars would be milk, fruits, and vegetables such as carrots, beets, squash, turnip and sweet potatoes.

How Rufus Beat Cancer ----------------------------

Here's another story I discovered...

Rufus was a ten year old Golden Retriever that was diagnosed with an inoperable cutaneous lymphoma.

Things did not look good...

Doctors gave poor Rufus just 6 months to live.

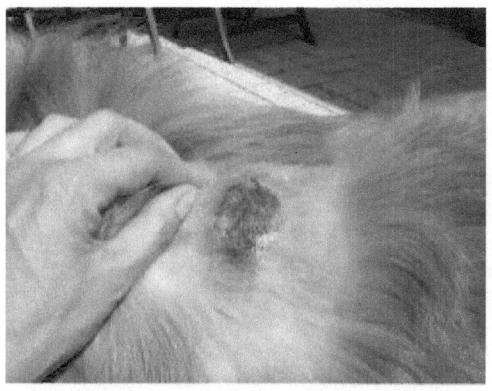

Dog's lymphoma tumor healing, week 2

But what happened blew everyone's mind

By simply adopting the healing "90 Day Canine Cancer Miracle Mix" you're about to see into Rufus's diet, his body obliterated his tumor in just six weeks.

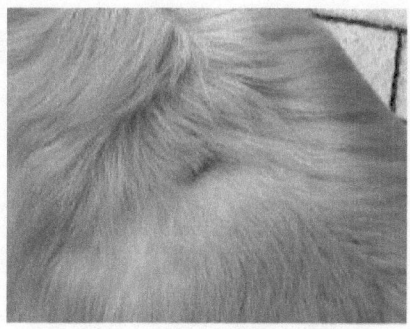

Dog's lymphoma tumor healing, week 6

Now keep in mind…

Rufus didn't follow any of the rules vets tell you to do…

He didn't go through torturous chemo…

He didn't suffer through radiation…

And he certainly didn't go through any expensive and painful surgery.

Instead, he simply followed this natural protocol we've been talking about.

Can you imagine?

Read on to see the exact "Mix" the Rufus used to heal.

THE SECOND RULE

Super Charge Your Dog's Health

As you learned in Rule #1, by cutting grains and sugars from your dog's diet, you are cutting cancer's main fuel source.

As cancer begins to starve, you can speed up your dog's healing time by supercharging his immune system.

You do this by adding antioxidants.

What are antioxidants?

Antioxidants are power substances found in plants that fight off damaging processes in your body.

Cancer epidemiologist John D. Potter of Seattle's Fred Hutchinson Cancer Research Center said,

> *"We're discovering a plethora of bioactive substances in plant foods."*

> *"These compounds seem to interact with every step in the cancer process, mostly slowing, stopping, or reversing them..."*

Yes, he said that the substances in plant foods could stop or reverse cancer.

Antioxidants fight free radicals, the wild carcinogens in your dog's body that are responsible for cancer.

And while everyone knows antioxidants are good for you... many have no idea they are good for your dog too.

Here are some of the most powerful ones for fighting cancer...

Suggested Dosage for Supplements

NOTE

Because of your dog's weight, fitness level, and health level, the dosage for supplements can vary drastically.

For that reason, we do not include doses for supplements that can be harmful to your dog if they are given too large a dose.

Consult with your veterinarian for proper dosing amounts

Vitamin C:

One of the most well know antioxidants is Vitamin C. It's found in most citrus fruits and can...

- Promote wound healing
- Strengthen blood vessels
- Maintain healthy skin
- Boost a weakened immune system,
- and prevent infections

There's also proof that Vitamin C aids dogs (and humans) with cancer.

In 39 people with terminal cancer, a study found that quality of life improved when combining IV and oral vitamin C (less pain, fatigue, nausea, and improved appetite).

Another study found that high doses of vitamin C killed cancer cells including lymphoma, mammary cancer, pheochromocytoma, kidney cancer, bladder cancer, lung cancer and glioblastoma cells.

Of course, many of these studies take place in a test tube, and your dog is a living breathing being. But just imagine if your dog got even a fraction of the benefits these studies say are possible? He could immediately start fighting off his cancers.

To sum up, when you are dealing with a life-threatening canine cancer, and your dog does not have calcium oxalate urinary stones, you should consider adding IV vitamin C to your dog's treatment plan.

Work with your vet to get IV vitamin C into your dog's diet. This is especially true if your dog's cancer is advanced.

World's Most Powerful Anti-Oxidant

But while vitamin C is good, there is one antioxidant shown by studies to be more powerful than all the rest.

In fact, a famous doctor calls it *"Natures' most powerful antioxidant."*

Because it's

— 6,000X MORE Powerful than Vitamin C

— 8000X more powerful than CoQ10, and

— 550X more powerful than Vitamin E and green tea

I'm talking about Astaxanthin.

It has very strong free radical scavenging abilities and helps protect cells, organs and tissues from oxidative damage.

Washington State University Published a study in the Journal of Animal Science on how Astaxanthin helps dogs.

What did they find?

"Dietary astaxanthin improved mitochondrial function in blood leukocytes, most likely by alleviating oxidative damage to cellular DNA and protein."

By adding astaxanthin, your dog's energy could drastically improve if you give him astaxanthin.

That's because mitochondria are the energy producers of a cell - what experts refer to as "tiny power plants."

When your dog is lethargic, there could be a mitochondrial problem. Diseases caused by mitochondrial problems in humans include autism, Parkinson's, Alzheimer's, and chronic fatigue syndrome.

Astaxanthin Study with Beagles

The WSU study involved both young and geriatric healthy female Beagles. The dogs were fed 20 mg of astaxanthin daily for 16 weeks. Fasting blood samples were taken at the start of the study, again at eight weeks, and again at the completion of the trial.

Mitochondrial function improved in both the young and elderly Beagles.

It's good for joints too

Astaxanthin provides antioxidants to parts of the body that don't normally receive a lot of antioxidant benefits. It can cross the blood-brain barrier and the blood-retina barrier. This means it can help reduce the potential for diseases of the central nervous system, the spinal cord, and the eye. Astaxanthin also supports immune function thanks to its high levels of beta-carotene.

Studies also show astaxanthin supports joint and muscle recovery after exercise and cardiovascular health in dogs and cats.

How much astaxanthin should you give your dog?

The first thing you should know is that your dog cannot overdose on astaxanthin.

But more does not always work better. There is a point of diminishing returns.

Start by feeding your dog the recommended dosage and add or decrease from there based on what you see.

Keep your vet informed on any supplements you plan to give your dog.

Arleigh Reynolds, a champion open class musher and top canine nutritionist recommends 2 – 4 mg (based on an average dog weight of 50 lbs.)

He says

"Of all the years I've spent studying sled dogs, especially antioxidants, I've found none better than Astaxanthin..."

"I've studied nutrition in sled dogs for close to 30 years and looked at lots of different ingredients and their effects. I can count on one hand, the things that actually make a difference in dog health over the course of a season and Astaxanthin is one of them."

Which astaxanthin product should you purchase?

I recommend Bioastin because of its production process. It's created by Nutrex in Hawaii. You can buy capsules for yourself at Costco or buy it in powder form on websites like Amazon. If you choose another product besides Bioastin, do research on the production process. Cheaper products may cut corners in the extraction process which makes astaxanthin's benefits useless.

Green Tea

Another great substance to feed your dog with cancer is green tea.

For starters, green tea is an excellent source of all sorts of antioxidants and Vitamins.

Research has shown Green Tea is packed with vitamin A, D, E, C, B, B5, H and K, manganese and other beneficial minerals such as zinc, chromium, and selenium to name just a few.

But Vitamins are just part of the story; fresh green tea leaves contain powerful antioxidants called polyphenols (specifically epigallocatechin gallate also known as EGCG).

This powerful catechin was found to be 25 to 100 times more potent than vitamins C and E.

It's also been shown to offer more antioxidant benefits than a serving of broccoli, spinach, carrots or strawberries.

In fact, according to veterinarians Steve Marsden, Shawn Messonnier and Cheryl Yuill:

"Green tea might be beneficial in any condition calling for the use of antioxidants. In humans, green tea is indicated as an antioxidant, an anti-cancer agent, and to lower blood cholesterol. Several tumor types are inhibited by green tea, including cancers of the stomach, gall bladder, prostate, uterus, lung, intestine, colon, rectum, and pancreas.

Green tea also inhibits breast cancer by binding to estrogen receptors, making it of potential value in the treatment of mammary gland cancer in small animals. Its comprehensive action against a variety of tumors in humans suggests green tea may provide the same benefits in animals.

Although they are absorbed into all body tissues, green tea catechins concentrate in the liver and digestive tract of dogs and laboratory animals, making it more likely they will be protective to these body regions."

In short, Green Tea is fantastic for your dog.

Here's a recipe on how best to give it to your dog from Dr. Becker DVM

Recipe for Organic Decaf Green Tea for Pets

1. Combine 1 liter (about 4 cups) of purified water and one tea bag or 1 tablespoon of loose tea leaves

2. Steep for 15 minutes

3. Remove the tea bag or use a strainer to remove the tea leaves

4. Store the tea in a covered, preferably glass pitcher in the fridge for up to three days

Add the following amounts of green tea to your pet's morning and evening meal:

- Cats, 1 tablespoon

- Small dogs, 1/8th cup

- Medium dogs, 1/4 to 1/2 cup

- Large dogs, 1/2 to 1 cup

Special Note: If your dog has been fasting or has not been eating well do NOT feed her green tea. Recent research has come out that reveals fasted dogs don't handle green tea well.

Arginine L

Arginine is an important amino acid for dogs.

Arginine can benefit the immune system and may influence tumor growth...
Although the optimal amount of arginine for dogs with cancer is unknown.

That's why it's important not to buy dog foods with arginine added.

You have no real idea how much is in there, and Arginine can easily be overdosed on.

Astragals Immunity Booster • Stimulates T-cell activity and raises white blood cell counts by improving liver function.

It boosts the body's defenses against disease and illness.

• Strengthens kidney function.
• Boosts energy level in dogs with serious diseases like cancer.

Prescribed for pets with chronic illnesses, infections, and cancer.

Because this works on the immune system, do not use this herb on your dog if they have an autoimmune disease.

Check first with your veterinarian.

Cats Claw

Cat's claw is a Peruvian herb that has recently been found to possess not only immune enhancing properties, but also antioxidant, anti-inflammatory, and anti-tumor properties.

It was first popularized by the German natural scientist Arturo Brell, who in 1926 migrated from Munich to Pozuzo, a small town founded by German colonists in the Peruvian rainforest.

Dr. Brell used cat's claw to treat his rheumatic pain.

He later treated another German colonist, Luis Schuler, who had been diagnosed with terminal lung cancer.
After other therapies had failed, Mr. Schuler began consuming cat's claw root tea three times a day.

He improved remarkably, and one year later was apparently free of cancer.

This fantastic herb is used for all types of conditions including arthritis, dermatitis, urinary infections, and of course cancer.

Enzymes

Human studies in athletes showed the enzymes dramatically improved healing time.

Other studies in humans showed enzymes taken with antibiotics increased how well the antibiotics work.

And studies in dogs are just as successful.

Enzymes break down protein and normally act as a digestive aid but they've also been shown to break down inflammation and speed up healing.

In 2002, Beverly Cappel, DVM, a holistic veterinarian in Chestnut Ridge, New York conducted a double-blind placebo-controlled crossover study of an enzyme supplement in the care and management of canine arthritis.

Dogs in the study stopped limping soon after the study started and owners noted they started acting like young dogs again.

Enzymes have therapeutic potential although limited approval in the United States.

L-asparaginase is probably the most valuable therapeutic modality for the treatment of lymphoma and leukemia in animals and people.

Recent studies have proven that enzymes help treat cancer patients, but veterinarians and researchers still don't know why.

One hypothesis is that these enzymes eliminate harmful pathogens in the body and therefore speed up healing.

Coenzyme Q10

This is an enzyme made by the body and found in the membranes of many tissues.

CoQ10 is a strong antioxidant and has a powerful effect on the immune system.

And that's important because it's been shown dog's with cancer have lower levels of CoQ10.

There is good evidence too that CoQ10 can actually increase cancer survival times.

But it's not just cancer, CoQ10 can help to protect your dog's heart and help lower blood pressure and help with repair incidental damage.

CoQ10 is especially good at reducing cardiotoxicity (toxicity to the heart) which occur as a side effect of a chemotherapy drug known as doxorubicin (Adriamycin).

Lena McCullough, DVM recommends dosing at, CoEnzyme Q10 at 200mg per day for dogs and 50mg per day for cats and smaller dogs.

Omega 3 Fatty Acids

Provide anti-inflammatory benefits that are especially important for dogs with cancer and may prevent the weight loss that can lead to cancer cachexia.

Many Omega 3s can become rancid in warm air. Refrigerate Omega 3s and use your supply within a few weeks of opening the bottle.

Typically, a dog with a raw, grass-fed meat diet, free of grains doesn't need much Omega 3 supplements.

Before adding Omega 3s, consider getting rid of grains and any vegetable oils in your dog's diet.

Why?

A review in the online journal BMJ showed that while eating more fish reduced stroke and other diseases in humans, no such benefit came from fish oil supplements.

In another study, the good fats under the Omega 3 label (DHA and EPA) werenabsorbed far better into the body after six weeks of salmon consumption versus fish oil supplements.

So maybe giving your dog fish is a better idea than giving him fish oil. Talk to your vet.

Symptoms of lack of Omega 3s -

- fatigues easily
- dry coat
- dry/flaky/itchy skin
- brittle nails
- joint pain

Important tip for Omega 3 Fatty Acids:

Check your dog's stool to make sure they are absorbing the Omega 3s. If the stool is oily, the Omega 3s are not being absorbed. Try a different product or giving your dog a smaller amount

Milk Thistle

Protects the liver and may prevent liver toxicity as a result of chemotherapy.

Speak to your veterinarian before giving your dog milk thistle.

It does stimulate the liver, and it's important not to over-stimulate the liver.

Milk thistle is well-known for its treatment of liver disease.

Do not use in pregnant animals.

Long term use in normal animals may result in depressed liver function unless a chronic liver disease is present.

It is not recommended to use milk thistle to prevent liver disease.

This holistic health remedy is most commonly used to detoxify a dog's liver.

If your dog has liver problems, this plant can help. It's even said to reduce the growth of cancer cells.

As an Antioxidant, milk thistle can improve recovery from infections, is useful following vaccinations and drug therapies.

Research on this herbal remedy isn't conclusive. Nevertheless, use of this ancient colorful flower seems very promising.

It is safe for use in dogs, in reasonable amounts but is NOT recommended as a daily supplement.

As Pat said March of 2016

"Ask your vet to prescribe milk thistle. My dog has Cushing's syndrome, and
that really damages the liver. My vet gave him milk thistle daily for two weeks.

Now he takes one tablet every 2-3 days for the rest of his life. Only 4 or 5 days
after starting, he became more like his old self. He's eating well and has a
renewed zest for life. I swear by it."

What it does: This flower contains a flavonoid called Silymarin which helps to release toxins which congregate in the liver. Plus, it helps cells to regenerate so can be an immunity booster.

Best used for: Liver Treatment

Heartworm (heartworm damages the organs). Milk thistle can be highly beneficial to dogs with heartworm and is the natural option to using chemically laced tick or flea prevention.

Milk Thistle to stop poisoning (contact vet)

If your dog ingests poisonous mushrooms, providing this herb may greatly detoxify their system. It can also treat things like lead poisoning and many other cases of poison or toxicities.

Other Milk Thistle Uses: Inflammatory bowel disease, digestive problems, skin problems caused by liver disease, cancer, bacterial infections, and inflammation

A Superfood for Dogs

Another supplement to use to increase the supply of vitamins and minerals to your dog is an all-natural, wholly absorbable, biologically available super green food called spirulina.

Spirulina is a freshwater, blue-green algae that is densely packed with fully absorbable protein. It contains a full spectrum of amino acids that absorb rapidly into your pet's bloodstream.

Spirulina is about 60 percent protein in its natural form, so it contains more protein ounce-for-ounce than meat. It is also a source of fatty acids, antioxidants, and phytonutrients. It is a wonderful whole food for pets.

Dr. Karen Becker uses Spirulina with her own pets and patients and has even published a book on the benefits. According to her:

> When an animal is starving or debilitated by a wound or disease, the gastrointestinal tract shuts down. Because Spirulina is composed of wholly absorbable nutrients – vitamins, amino acids, fatty acids, antioxidants and phytonutrients – it can be passively assimilated by the GI tract. In other words, an animal's body doesn't have to work hard to absorb all the wonderful nutrients in Spirulina.
>
> When food is reintroduced to a starving animal, it must be done very slowly. Spirulina is perfect for this application and prevents the body from going into shock when it is starved for nutrients.

The maximum dose to give your dog is 1 to 2 tablespoons for a 45 lb dog. Start by giving your dog a small amount and slowly increasing the dosage over time based on your dog's results.

Lastly, no matter how sick your dog gets, don't forget about sunlight. No, I'm not talking about just supplementing with Vitamin D. Your dog needs real sunlight. That's because the UV rays help your body generate nitric oxide the most important chemicals in the body to promote proper circulation.

Success Story Highlight --------------

Mary Never Gave Up on Ted

Ted was motionless. For nine weeks, mass celled cancer tumors ravaged his body.

Veterinarians washed their hands of his case. Not willing to give up without a fight, Mary, his owner, was desperate for a solution.

So she tried "The Mix" you're about to read about right now.

Within two days, she could see a change in Ted, his spunk returning. At day 14, one of his open tumors became a scab. In six weeks, his tumor had disappeared.

To the shock of the veterinary world, more than eight years later, Ted is a healthy, happy dog.

Thanks to Johanna Budwig and her work creating "The Mix" that makes the 90 Day Canine Cancer Cure possible...

The scientific world is finally acknowledging what a small community of natural healers has known for over 60 years...

Cancer is not the end of the road.

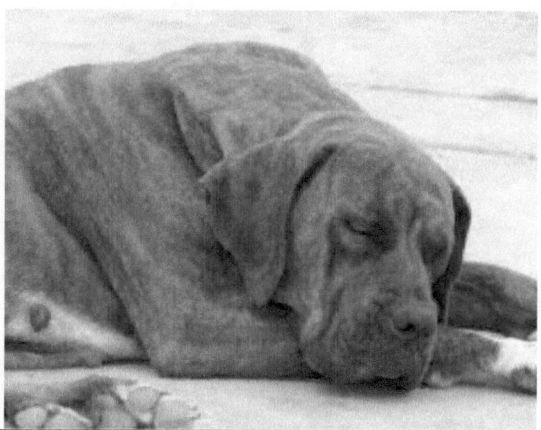

Your first two steps were to cut out grains and sugars and to use antioxidants to boost your dog's immune system. But this third and final step is the most CRITICAL.

Let me warn you, while it may seem too easy to be effective; this final step could be the one thing that cures your dog's cancer for good.

THE THIRD RULE

Oxygenate Cells with the "Power Mix"

Don't be fooled by its simplicity. What you're about to see is incredibly effective.

The Independent Cancer Research Foundation concluded, "it stops the spread of cancer and kills cancer cells."

And Dr. Roehm M.D., a world renowned oncologist calls this treatment, "By far and away the most successful anti-cancer treatment of its kind in the world."

This step alone has healed countless dogs from late stage cancer.

Dogs so sick they'd been completely written off by mainstream medicine.

Why is it so effective?

Because after you've cut off cancers fuel, and boosted your dog's immune system in steps one and two, now it's time to oxygenate your dog's cells.

What happens is, cancer starves your cells of oxygen, and they begin to die. But oxygenating your dog's cells is actually very easy, as Dr. Johanna Budwig discovered.

It has to do with combining a few simple foods you might already have at your home right now into something called the "Power Mix."

Making the "Mix" is simple. You just need a few ingredients.

1. Unfiltered flax seed oil (Barleans brand is a good choice available at whole foods and other health food stores.)

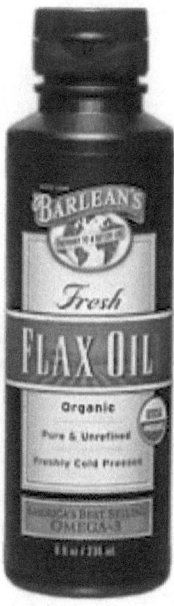

Be sure to buy the regular flax seed oil and not the high lignans. We'll be adding our own to this mix in the form of freshly ground seeds.

2. Low fat (less than 2%) organic cottage cheese

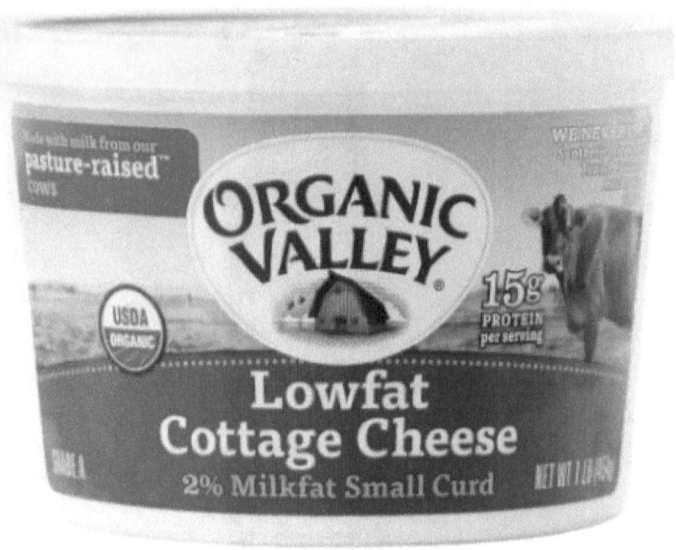

3. A hand blender or emulsifier

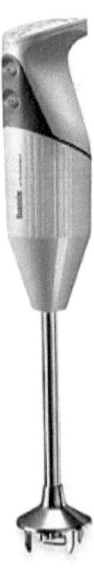

4. Fresh flax seeds

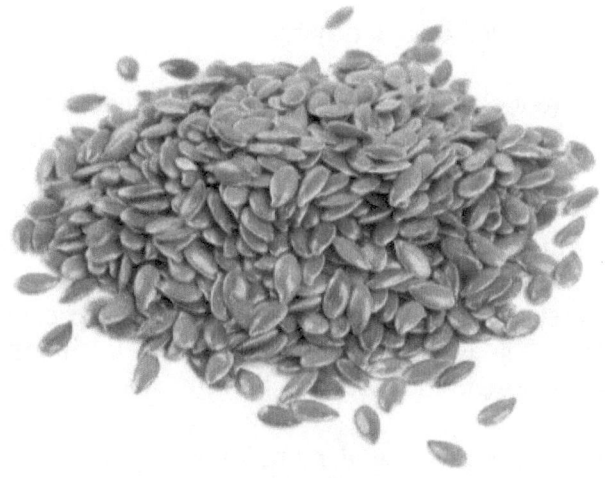

5. Grinder

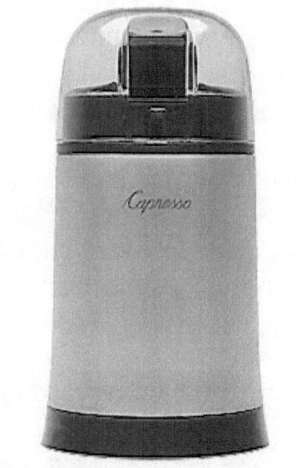

--Dosage: 1 part flax oil to 2 parts cottage cheese.

For treatment of cancer: feed your dog the following mix twice a day.

For prevention: Feed once a day.

The ratio we are looking at of FLAX OIL to cottage cheese is 1:2 (1 tablespoon of flax oil to 2 tablespoons of cottage cheese).

If your dog is **25 pounds** or under, he should consume 1 ½ tablespoons of flaxseed oil to 3 tablespoons of cottage cheese daily.

You should break this up into two meals...¾ of a tablespoon of flax oil and with 1 ½ tablespoons of cottage cheese in the morning and repeat the same dose in the evening.

If your dog is **50 pounds** or under aim for three tablespoons of flaxseed oil and six tablespoons of cottage cheese spread out over the day. (1 1/2 teaspoons of flaxseed oil and three tablespoons cottage cheese in the morning and the same dose again in the evening.)

If you have a large dog up to (100 pounds), your goal is six tablespoons of FLAX OIL per day with 12 tablespoons of cottage cheese. (3 tablespoons flax seed oil and six tablespoons cottage cheese in the morning and the same dose again in the evening.)

**Word of caution, start slow and build up to the full dose.

That's because if you immediately start with the full dose, you run the risk of irritating your dog's stomach and causing diarrhea and intestinal discomfort.

We recommend you start with half the recommended dose for the first week to see how your dog responds. If your dog shows no sign of problems slowly increase the dose each week until you reach the recommended levels.

Making the Mix

A Step by Step Guide

Step 1-- Begin by blending the organic flax seed oil with organic cottage cheese for roughly a minute.

Do not use a blender. It won't mix it up properly and give us the oxygen we are looking for. Instead, use a hand emulsifier. (See image below.)

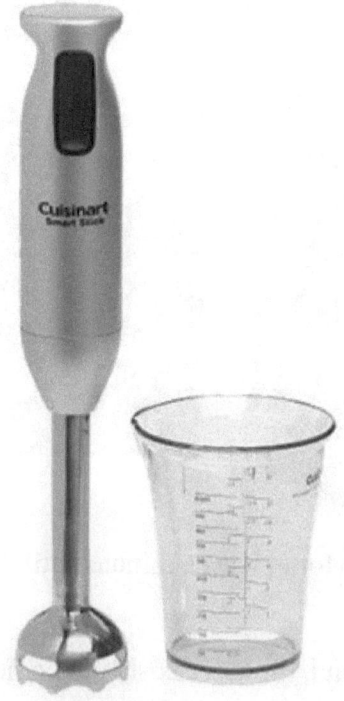

After a minute of blending there should be no oil left on top of the mix and it should have the consistency of a rich whipped cream or smoothie.

You know you are done when you can hold a spoonful of the mix upside down, and no oil escapes.

Remember--mix the flax seed oil and the cottage cheese together first with no other ingredients added.

This allows for the proper bonding to take place to make this mix effective as
possible.

Step 2-- Add in 1-2 tablespoons (depending on the size of your dog) of fresh brown organic flax seeds to a coffee bean grinder.

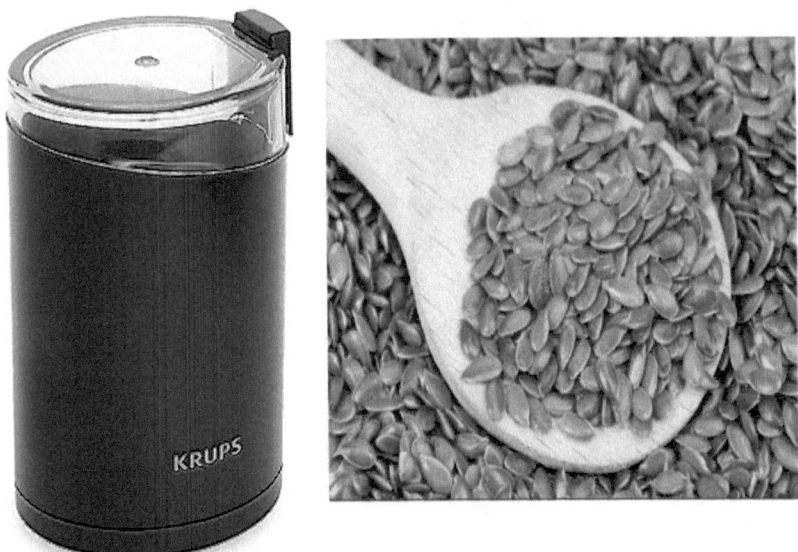

Grind these seeds for at least a minute until they are ground into small bits.

After a proper grind, these seeds should come out nice and fluffy.

Step 3-- Add the ground flax seeds to the flax oil and cottage cheese mix and stir with a spoon.

Step 4-- Feed this mix to your dog twice a day. You can either stir this mix into his regular food, or you can give it to him after his meal as a treat.

Things to keep in mind

--Do not pre make this mix. Once flax seeds are ground up, they begin to oxygenate very quickly. So to maximize the healing potential of the mix be sure and have your dog consume the product within 20 minutes of making it.

--Try to use only organic ingredients if possible.

How to tell if this Protocol is working

While there are no sure signs without a doctor's diagnosis, yet there are three common ones we see to indicate the 90-day protocol is working:

1. Appetite returning: Sick dogs don't like to eat. When a dog is on the mend, he'll make rapid strides to tell you he's feeling better.

2. Look in your dog's eyes. The eyes are a great source of information about a pup's health because they're connected to both the vascular and neurologic systems. A healthy pup will have clear alert eyes. Watch carefully for changes.

3. Energy levels are picking up. If your dog is up and running around and wanting to walk and play...that's a very good sign that "the mix" is doing its job.

Important Information about Flax Oil

Only use Flax Oil from the refrigerated section of your health food store. Never use capsules, flakes or flax oil from the shelves. It must be refrigerated and check the expiration date to make sure it has not expired. I would not use High Lignan Flax Oil because the taste is not clean and you cannot tell if it is rancid. They have left the husk from the processing of the seeds in the bottom of the bottle, leaving less product. You want good clean tasting oil, and no flavoring added as some oils are doing.

Consume "the Mix" immediately.

Do not add anything to the mixture until AFTER it is mixed.

We recommend using the immersion (stick or wand like) mixer for the Flax Seed Oil and Cottage Cheese.

The mixture is correctly mixed if you can hold a spoonful upside down for a few moments and the mixture does not fall out.

What people are saying…

"Must buy for Dog Cancer Patient's!"

I wish this were available several years ago before I lost 7 dogs to cancer, despite surgeries. I adopted two senior golden retriever rescues last year and when I took them to the vet, got the dreaded cancer diagnosis again! I'm actually watching the male's tumors shrink. They both are happier and more active. Worth every penny. Everything needed to supplement their meals is available on Amazon.

"What a difference!"

I bought this after a bone biopsy on our dog came back as bone cancer. We decided against amputation and no chemo. I have been following the suggestions in this book for feeding and supplements for 30 days now. My dog is 90% back to her old self. She wants to play fetch outside, has an appetite again, talks to us when we come home. What a difference! If it weren't for her one weak back leg, you would never know she has cancer. I would highly recommend this book!

Special Note--When **Not** to use this protocol. Due to the nature of flaxseed oil if your dog is close to surgery or currently on blood thinning medication it is best to avoid this nutritional protocol and consult with your veterinarian.

How to Feed our Dog after they are Cured

When your dog has cancer, you want to pick foods that are highly palatable and has lots of kcal/cup of food. A sick dog doesn't need to eat as much to meet its energy needs. Look for a diet where 30-50 percent of the calories come from a good quality protein source, 50-60 percent of the calories come from fat, and the rest of the calories come from carbohydrates. There are commercially prepared foods available for dogs on cancer treatment, but you will need to ask your veterinarian to order them for you.

Although research on every kind of cancer hasn't been done yet, many types of cancer cells feed on the sugars in carbohydrates, high fructose fruits, and starchy veggies; however, most cancer cells cannot feed on good fats. The idea with a preventative diet, then, is to keep your pet's carb content low, while keeping protein and good fats high. This generally means staying away from traditional carb-based grain kibbles and moving towards something more whole-foods based.

A general, suggested breakdown is:

Dogs: 50% protein (fish or poultry is best), 50% veggies (dark leafy greens, carrots, broccoli, zucchini, and green beans are good choices).

Is Your Dog's Water Making Him Sicker?

Depending on where you live, the water might carry more toxins than you realize. Although it might taste fine, and everyone in the house seems fine, over time, the build-up of chemicals can lead to serious health problems, including cancer.

To combat this, offer your pet filtered water that you change frequently. Also, be sure to use glass or ceramic bowls, so toxins from plastic don't leach into the water. Yes, that means using store-bought water from plastic bottles is a no-no as well.

Weight

One other dietary issue needs mentioning, and that is weight management. Overweight pets are at increased risk of many diseases, such as arthritis, diabetes, and heart disease as well as cancer. Food does not equal love; your pet would rather have quality time with you than a big dinner or a few extra treats. Even more importantly, fat doesn't just sit there quietly; it produces inflammatory mediators that can contribute to tumor formation. Keeping your pet at an ideal weight is an essential part of a healthy lifestyle.

For additional information about the benefits of fresh food and a healthy diet, please read our article: *What You Need to Know About Your Pet's Food.*

"Any cancer prevention or treatment program begins with diet. Nothing will go farther in promoting health than a balanced, home-prepared diet of fresh, preferably organic, whole foods."

Don't allow your dog to become overweight. Studies prove that restricting a number of calories an animal eats prevents and delays the progression of tumor development across species, including canines.

Fewer calories cause the cells of the body to block tumor growth, whereas too many calories can lead to obesity, and obesity is closely linked to increased cancer risk in humans. There is a connection between too much glucose, increased insulin sensitivity, inflammation, and oxidative stress – all factors in obesity – and cancer.

It's important to remember that fat doesn't just sit on your pet's body harmlessly. It produces inflammation that can promote tumor development. **Feed an anti-inflammatory diet.** Anything that creates or promotes inflammation in the body increases the risk for cancer. Current research suggests cancer is actually a chronic inflammatory disease. The inflammatory process creates an environment in which abnormal cells proliferate.

Cancer cells require the glucose in carbohydrates to grow and multiply, so you want to limit or eliminate that cancer energy source. Carbs to remove from your pet's diet include processed grains, fruits with fructose, and starchy vegetables like potatoes. Keep in mind that all dry pet food contains some form of starch. It may be grain-free, but it can't be starch-free because it's not possible to manufacture kibble without using some type of starch.

Cancer cells generally can't use dietary fats for energy, so appropriate amounts of good quality fats are nutritionally healthy for dogs.

Another major contributor to inflammatory conditions is a diet too high in omega-6 fatty acids and too low in **omega-3s**. Omega-6s increase inflammation while the omega-3s do the reverse. Processed pet food is typically loaded with omega-6 fatty acids and deficient in omega-3s.

A healthy diet for your pet – one that is anti-inflammatory and anti-cancer – consists of real, whole foods, preferably raw. It should be high in high-quality protein, including muscle meat, organs, and bone. It should include moderate amounts of animal fat and high levels of EPA and DHA (omega-3 fatty acids), a few fresh cut veggies and a bit of fruit.

This species-appropriate diet is high in moisture content and contains no grains or starches. I also recommend adding a vitamin/mineral supplement and a few beneficial supplements like probiotics, digestive enzymes, and super green foods.

Reduce or eliminate your dog's exposure to toxins. These include chemical pesticides like **flea and tick preventives, lawn chemicals** (weed killers, herbicides, etc.), tobacco smoke, **flame retardants**, and **household cleaners** (detergents, soaps, cleansers, dryer sheets, room deodorizers).

Because we live in a toxic world and avoiding all chemical exposure is nearly impossible, offer a periodic detoxification protocol to your pets.

Allow your dog to remain intact (not neutered or spayed), at least until the age of 18 months to two years. Studies have linked spaying and neutering to increasing cancer rates in dogs. A 2002 study established an increased risk of osteosarcoma in both male and female Rottweilers neutered or spayed before the age of one year. Another study showed the risk of bone cancer in neutered or spayed large purebred dogs was twice that of intact dogs.

Refuse unnecessary vaccinations. Vaccine protocols should be tailored to minimize risk and maximize protection, taking into account the breed, background, nutritional status and overall vitality of the dog. The protocol I follow with healthy puppies is to provide a single parvo and distemper vaccine at or before 12 weeks, and the second set after 14 weeks. I then titer (ask your vet to run titers at a lab that uses the IFA method) two weeks after the last set, and if the dog has been successfully immunized, he is protected for life.

If titer tests indicate vaccine levels are low (which would be incredibly unlikely), I recommend a booster for only the specific virus or viruses that titered low, and only for those to which the animal has a real risk of exposure. I do not use or recommend combination vaccines (six to eight viruses in one injection), which is the standard yearly booster at many veterinary practices.

http://www.onlynaturalpet.com/holistic-healthcare-library/food-diet---general/4/what-you-need-to-know-about-your-pets-food.aspx

More Tips to Boost Your Dog's Immune System

Warning: If your pet is on chemotherapy or is immunosuppressed, you should not feed a raw diet.

Sources of Good Fats and other supplements that can be added to your dog's food to boost their immune system:

— Flax oil (1 teaspoon per 20 pounds daily)

— Olive oil (1 teaspoon per 20 pounds daily)

— Coconut oil (1 teaspoon per 10 pounds daily--might have to start with smaller dose and work up)

— Fish oil (1000 mg per 10-20 pounds daily)

— Turmeric (less than 1 tablespoon daily)

— Garlic (1/2 clove for dogs under 40 pounds, 1 clove for dogs over 40 pounds, daily for 5 days, then rest for 2. Cats should not get garlic.)

— Milk Thistle (200 mg per 10 pounds, daily)

— Spirulina

— Chlorella

The Truth about Chemotherapy

When all else fails, is chemotherapy safe?

The dirty secret about chemotherapy is that not only is it expensive painful and causes horrendous side effects…it also flat out doesn't work.

Unbelievable? Perhaps.

But a quick look at the numbers shows that chemotherapy cures 2% of all patients.

And the sad fact is doctors know it. Chemotherapy *has always been developed from toxic, poisonous chemicals, right? So, there has always been a fine line between administering a "therapeutic dose" and killing the cancer patient. Many doctors step over that line.*

But don't take it from me!

Here's what Dr. Allen Levin says about this topic: *"Most cancer patients in this country die of chemotherapy. Chemotherapy does not eliminate breast, colon, or lung cancers. This fact has been documented for over a decade, yet doctors still use chemotherapy for these tumors."*

Just think about it…

To put it plainly, the treatment kills them before cancer kills them. As a matter of fact, the chemotherapy drug 5FU is sometimes referred to by doctors as "5 feet under" because of its deadly side effects. For most adult cancers, the typical best case scenario is that the "Big 3" buys a little time. In a worst case scenario, you will die from the treatment rather than the disease.

In his book, *When Healing Becomes a Crime*, Kenny Ausubel notes that in a trial on a chemotherapy drug tested for leukemia, a whopping 42% of the patients died directly from the toxicity of the chemotherapy drug!

Here are the facts. In 1942, Memorial Sloan-Kettering Cancer Center quietly began to treat breast cancer with these mustard gas derivatives. No one was cured. Chemotherapy trials were also conducted at Yale around 1943 where 160 patients were treated. Again, no one was cured.

According to Dr. John Diamond, M.D., "A study of over 10,000 patients shows clearly that chemotherapy's supposedly strong track record with Hodgkin's disease (lymphoma) is actually a lie. Patients who underwent chemotherapy were 14 times more likely to develop leukemia and 6 times more likely to develop cancers of the bones, joints, and soft tissues than those patients who did not undergo chemotherapy."

Dr. Glenn Warner, who died in 2000, was one of the most highly qualified cancer specialists in the United States. He used alternative treatments on his cancer patients with great success. On the treatment of cancer in this country, he said: "We have a multi-billion dollar industry that is killing people, right and left, just for financial gain. Their idea of research is to see whether two doses of this poison is better than three doses of that poison."

Dr. Alan C. Nixon, past president of the American Chemical Society, writes, "As a chemist trained to interpret data, it is incomprehensible to me that physicians can ignore the clear evidence that chemotherapy does much, much more harm than good." And according to Dr. Charles Mathe, French cancer specialist, "…if I contracted cancer, I would never go to a standard cancer treatment center. Only cancer victims who live far from such centers have a chance."

Yet day after day, year after year, the Cancer Industry continues to put these toxic chemicals into the bodies of cancer patients. And the patients let them do it, even volunteering for new "guinea pig" studies, simply because someone with a degree from a school of disease (also known as medical school) told them it was their "only option." It costs lots of money for them to poison the body of cancer patients, and the patients gladly pay it. Sadly, some people will spend six figures a year poisoning their bodies because their "doctor told them to do it."

The truth is chemotherapy makes money for big corporations. Do your research before going down this path.

REFERENCES

1. http://healthypets.mercola.com/sites/healthypets/archive/2012/03/05/common-cancer-for-pet-dogs-and-cats-mast-cell-tumors.aspx

2. http://www.petsafe.net/learn/pet-food-the-good-the-bad-and-the-healthy

3. www.WholisticVet.com

4. http://indiantime.net/story/2014/03/27/News/Jenna-Herne%2C-LVT-Volunteers-for-Iditarod-Race-in-Alaska/13405.html

5. http://pets.webmd.com/dogs/dog-teeth-care

6. http://akitarescue.com/Budwig%20Formula.htm